IS AMERICAN PSYCHIATRIC

PRACTICE DISEASED

BEYOND RECOVERY?

To my children, Ida, a political science professor, and Jesse, a medical student about to specialize in psychiatry: keep up your critical thinking

CONTENTS

ACKNOWLEDGMENTS

A big hug for my lovely wife, Devra, who helped, edited and supported me in writing this text.

INTRODUCTION

Psychiatric disorders are very common. Many start early in life, are chronic, and disrupt human development and functioning significantly. According to the World Health Organization, several mental illnesses are among the top ten disability causing problems in the world. Depression, with onset possible throughout the life cycle, is anticipated to be the second most frequent medical condition in the world by the year 2020, only surpassed by cardiovascular disease. Schizophrenia, with onset usually in the second or third decade of life, occurs in about one percent of the population worldwide, causing tremendous personal suffering, family problems and societal costs. Attention deficit hyperactivity disorder (ADHD) starts early in childhood and continues to affect approximately three to four percent of adults. Impairments in academic, occupational, and interpersonal functioning are well documented in this chronic condition. Anxiety disorders, addiction, and eating disorders are other examples of common mental health problems. Suicide, many times the result of a mental illness, is among the top causes of mortality in adolescents and young adults.

By and large, one in five persons will experience a significant psychiatric condition in their life time. This should not come as a surprise. Mental functioning is orchestrated by the brain, by far the most complex organ in the body.

Psychiatric problems are not only important because they disrupt normal human thinking and behavior, but also because they interact with other general medical conditions. For example, an intricate connection exists between heart disease and depression. On the one hand, it appears that chronic depression is a risk factor for cardiac problems in later life. On the other hand, when heart disease is accompanied by depression, the prognosis is more guarded and mortality is increased. The biological underpinnings of this interaction are beginning to be understood.

There is also a growing evidence base of the connection between depression and obesity, the modern day epidemic. Again, a bi-directional relationship may be present: depression leading to more weight gain, and obesity increasing depressive symptoms.

The relationship between mind and body is also apparent in the fact that patients with certain psychiatric disorders have a much higher incidence of obesity, type 2 diabetes mellitus, hypertension and cardiovascular disease. For example, in the U.S., persons with schizophrenia have a reduction in their life expectancy of 15 to 20 years, because of these associated health issues.

In developed and developing countries around the world, mental illness will increasingly demand attention as an important health determining variable.

It logically follows that psychiatric treatment should be readily available and of high quality. A growing understanding of the nature of psychiatric conditions should lead to better diagnosis and treatment. In this regard, the decade of the brain in the 1990's saw an explosion of research in the treatment of depression, anxiety, schizophrenia, substance abuse, attention deficit and other disorders. Large epidemiological studies mapped out the prevalence of mental illness in the community. Research in the biological mechanisms of normal and abnormal psychological functioning grew exponentially. New treatments came about. Several new classes of psychotropic medications became available. Evidence based psychotherapies, such as cognitive and interpersonal therapy, became the gold standard in the psychological treatment of a variety of conditions. Invasive procedures, such as deep brain stimulation, and non-invasive procedures, such as trans-cranial magnetic stimulation, were beginning to be studied for treatment of refractory patients with depression and obsessive compulsive disorder. Real world treatment outcome studies in schizophrenia, bipolar disorder, and depression were undertaken in the U.S. and Europe, producing large amounts of data. Current ongoing scientific inquiry focuses on genetic and epigenetic contributions to the etiology and physiology of psychiatric conditions, and may at some point in time bring personalized medicine to psychiatry.

In conclusion, there is much more to be studied, but there is a reasonable body of evidence available to guide psychiatric interventions.

Psychiatrists, like other medical specialists, need to keep up with new developments in their field. This is a daunting task. Research is increasing rapidly, but, not infrequently, there is a problem applying the findings of controlled studies to the real world. For example, neuro-imaging is identifying the brain parts and nerve pathways involved in anxiety disorders, depression, and schizophrenia, but there is no use for these techniques in the clinic as of yet. The mapping of the human genome made it possible to identify certain genes as factors to increase the risk for certain mental illnesses, but few genetic tests are ready to be used in the clinic. To help clinicians wade through the enormous amount of information, different organizations have created guidelines on the diagnosis and treatment of many mental health conditions. These documents are periodically revised and updated. Diagnosis and treatment of mental illness should reflect these current evidence based guidelines.

So how is contemporary psychiatry, as it is practiced in the community across the United States, doing? Are U.S. psychiatrists indeed keeping up with new data in their field? Are guidelines being followed? Are newly available medications used appropriately? Is the interaction with other medical conditions considered in the treatment of mental illness?

I have written this book to provide an inside view. It is important to keep in mind that the observations contained in this text are not the result of a scientific study, but based upon my personal experiences during the last 30 years, in a variety of treatment settings: academic medical centers, general hospitals, private practices, community clinics, residential treatment programs, forensic facilities and the like. This book is the account of only one psychiatrist, but the examples in the text are not based on local observations only. For the past 15 years, I have traveled to many hospitals and clinics and have spoken to many psychiatrists in different states of this country. Because of my travels, I am convinced the text shows the average standard of care in many psychiatric settings in the U.S.

At the end, it will be clear that this quality of care, as provided in many practices, is extremely low. I will try to provide a possible explanation why it has come to such a disastrous level. While doing so, real examples of the problems will be provided. An alarming erosion of any scientific standard will become apparent.

This book is not pointing the finger at every psychiatrist and every psychiatric clinic, but I believe problems are pervasive enough for real concern. And even though many other factors are playing a role in the deterioration of psychiatric care, it is ultimately the responsibility of the individual medical doctor to remain truthful to his or her medical mission: quality patient care, lifelong learning, practicing according to established standards, following risk management strategies, maintaining professionalism and ethical values.

Other factors that have undermined the quality of care will only be discussed briefly. Managed care companies, lawyers, and a society looking for magic pills and quick fixes, are factors interrelated with the central problem in American psychiatric practice.

Why did I write this book? To me, it appears that no one is paying attention to the day to day quality of care that many psychiatrists are providing. Although it is far from clear what will need to happen to turn this situation around, the first step is to provide an eye opener. Even if there is only one psychiatrist who reads the book and, as a result, improves his or her practice, many patients will benefit, and the book will have been worthwhile.

In the last two chapters, some ways to improve upon the current situation are presented. In the U.S., initiatives to enhance the quality of care in medicine are clearly underway, not just in psychiatry. But will these changes be sufficient for the mental health field? Personally, I do not believe so. Therefore, ultimately I offer a radical and controversial idea. The problem is indeed formidable, the solution elusive, but I continue to hope that the new generation of psychiatrists will improve this situation.

I also realize that I open myself up to a lot of criticism. I believe that the examples in the book speak for themselves, however. And while no one's practice of medicine is perfect, psychiatry, as a field, appears to be in need of some serious soul searching

CHAPTER 1: WHAT IS PSYCHIATRY?

Psychiatry is a medical specialty, like cardiology, neurology, surgery. In the United States, psychiatrists are medical doctors who have completed four years of undergraduate studies, four years of medical school, and at least four years of residency training. It is important to consider for a moment this long and intensive education. Medical school starts with the study of the basic sciences underlying normal and abnormal functioning of the human body: anatomy, histology, embryology, physiology, biochemistry, etc. Subsequently, different systems and their malfunctions are considered: the cardiovascular, musculoskeletal, gastro-intestinal, endocrinological, respiratory, metabolic and central nervous systems. Disease states and their treatments are learned while the application of this knowledge to the individual patient's situation is practiced. Medical students, including future psychiatrists, spend the last two years of their curriculum rotating through different services, such as internal medicine, surgery, pediatrics, obstetrics, neurology, psychiatry, etc.

In residency, newly graduated doctors work closely under the supervision of medical specialists within a certain area to treat patients, while honing their diagnostic and treatment skills. Residency programs have a minimum duration of three years, for example in internal medicine or pediatrics. Psychiatry residencies are four years long. During the first year, psychiatric residents spend four months in internal medicine and two months in neurology. The remainder is spent in psychiatric settings under the supervision of psychiatrists.

Medical training is a very intellectual exercise: physicians need to store enormous amounts of information in their memory, while using differential diagnostic thinking skills as their ultimate tool.

Diagnoses are remembered as prototypes, against which the individual patient's signs and symptoms are compared. A good examination will identify positive and negative findings, which will guide the physician in determining what prototype diagnosis resembles the patient's condition. Further testing, such as blood tests, electrophysiological tests, imaging studies, can help validate the physician's diagnostic reasoning by excluding certain conditions and confirming others.

Specialties like internal medicine and pediatrics use the critical thinking skills as their main diagnostic devices. They are considered "cognitive" specialties, in contrast to surgical ones where other skills are more important. What about psychiatry? It is clearly a cognitive specialty as well. But the medical specialty of psychiatry is quite unique in that it has no objective tests to confirm or dispel a diagnosis. There is no blood test, imaging machine, or tissue biopsy that will identify an existing mental illness. That means that there is no feedback on the diagnostic thinking of the psychiatrist. This fact is at the core of the problem in psychiatric practice, as will be shown later. At the same time, psychiatric disorders are brain problems, with the brain being an enormously complex organ. It is still pretty much a black box: quite mysterious in its function and dysfunction. So, psychiatrists are dealing with the most complex organ in the animal kingdom, without any objective tests results to be their guides.

Psychiatry is the most cognitive of specialties because almost the entire examination happens at a verbal level. Critical thinking skills are by and large the only diagnostic tool that psychiatrists can use. But psychiatrists spend on average only four months in internal medicine and two months in neurology during their four years of psychiatric residency. Honing their critical differential diagnostic skills after that period depends on learning solely from other psychiatrists. While doctors in training for other cognitive specialties spend three years in residency, receiving continuous feedback on their diagnostic abilities through a variety of tests, future psychiatrists spend only six months in such an environment. This may be a problem, as will become evident later in this text.

Neurology is the other medical specialty dealing with the central nervous system. However, neurology concerns itself most with the sensori-motor system, not the brain parts involved in mood, thinking and behavior, like psychiatry. Medical science has made significant progress in creating objective tests to identify problems in these basic sensori-motor brain parts: EEG, CT scan, MRI, electrophysiological studies and brain biopsies are examples of diagnostic tools in neurology. But psychiatry has not reached this level of sophistication in its study of the brain's more intricate electrochemical circuits underlying the most human qualities of emotional and cognitive functioning.

While some minor progress is being made in objectifying findings in mental illness, the day to day practice of psychiatric medicine rests entirely upon the cognitive skills of the physician without feedback from other disciplines like radiology, pathology, or microbiology. In this regard, findings of the psychiatric examination, which is done entirely through verbal questions, need to be documented in a comprehensive manner. This again raises a serious problem in psychiatric practice, which will be discussed.

Another aspect of the medical profession cannot be ignored: the need for lifelong learning. At the end of medical school, all doctors take an oath, based on the original oath of Hippocrates from several thousand years ago. Every oath contains the promise that physicians will continue to study the art and science of medicine throughout their careers. The explosion in scientific knowledge, the limitations of the human memory, and the unavoidable maintenance of old habits, create this requirement for continuous theoretical and experiential learning. This need may be even more important in a field like psychiatry, where no independent confirmation of one's thinking is available. But are psychiatrists following their oath?

Psychiatrists are dealing with the most complex organ in the body without the aid of any objective tests and with a minimal amount of training in differential diagnostic thinking where feedback is available. These facts should lead to meticulous documentation and an investment in ongoing education.

CHAPTER II: THE PROBLEM IN PSYCHIATRY: LACK OF CORRECTIVE FEEDBACK

Let's consider the following scenario: a 50 year old man presents to his primary care physician with complaints of chest pain. After a rudimentary examination, the physician concludes the patient is having a heart attack and sends him to the nearest emergency room. A thorough evaluation is done in the emergency department. The patient's electrocardiogram is entirely normal. Laboratory results, reasonably specific for myocardial damage, come back normal as well. The patient even undergoes a coronary angiogram which shows no occlusion of any coronary artery. After further tests, it is concluded that the patient's chest pain was related to acid reflux from the stomach into the esophagus. All results are sent to the primary care physician.

This physician is getting feedback on his work: his reasoning that the patient had a heart attack was wrong. The physician got this corrective feedback from numerous sources: the more thorough history and physical examination of the emergency room doctor, the ECG, the blood work, and the angiogram imaging test. The next time a similar situation presents itself, the thinking process of this physician will have been shaped by this experience: a more thorough history, a more extensive physical examination, and even some objective tests may be done in the office. Over years of practice, through the process of corrective feedback, this physician's memory templates of different diagnoses will be changed, his differential diagnostic thinking will be enhanced, and his care to patients will be improved.

This process occurs multiple times per day for most physicians. When a patient complains of headaches, the doctor may think they are due to hypertension. But upon measuring a normal blood

9

pressure in the patient, the physician will need to redo his diagnostic assessment. Many times, concrete numbers, pictures or values guide this re-assessment of the patient's condition. Patients can use numbers to guide their health status as well: blood pressure, cholesterol, blood sugar, triglycerides, hemoglobin A1c, PSA, are all tests with specific numbers and guidelines that physicians and patients can use to monitor their health and treatment.

No such corrective feedback process exists in psychiatry. To this date, there is not one test that can confirm or revoke a diagnosis of mental illness. An objective number showing how depressed a patient really is does not exist. There is no instrument showing how strong hallucinatory voices dominate a person's experience. There is no panic anxiety blood test. There is no reliable computer test for attention deficit hyperactivity disorder. This is a far reaching problem. The biggest issue comes down to the patients: they may be misdiagnosed, they may receive the wrong treatments, and they may become demoralized with the varied opinions they receive from different doctors.

I see many patients whose diagnoses have changed several times, with the only intervening variable being the different psychiatrists who have seen the patient.

Recently, I saw someone I had diagnosed with schizophrenia ten years ago, based on pervasive auditory hallucinations, severe paranoid and bizarre delusions (convinced that people were aliens trying to poison him; subatomic particle waves generated by aliens were meant to control his behavior and thinking), negative symptoms of schizophrenia (flat affect, poverty of speech, lack of motivation) and cognitive symptoms (poor retention of information). Over the past ten years, he had been followed by two other psychiatrists, who also diagnosed him with schizophrenia (or at least did not see the need to change the original diagnosis). When I saw him again, he presented in a very similar condition, although he was refusing to take antipsychotic medication. Shortly thereafter, unbeknownst to me, he was involuntarily committed to a psychiatric unit for homicidal ideation toward specific individuals. After 10 days in the hospital, the patient was released with a discharge diagnosis of major depressive disorder!

What happened here? How is this possible? Who is right? And most importantly, how is this affecting the patient? Many questions can be raised about this scenario: did the patient not reveal his delusional thoughts in the hospital? Were his negative symptoms of schizophrenia interpreted as depressive symptoms? Why did the hospital not contact me to coordinate care? Was the correct treatment provided despite the differing diagnoses?

This case report exemplifies the core problem in psychiatry: no one can do an objective test to see what problem the patient really has. Even if the hospital and I had communicated (some form of feedback), there could still have been disagreement over the patient's problem. Medical and psychiatric conditions share symptoms. Fever happens in viral and bacterial infections, but objective tests can differentiate the two types of infections. Lack of motivation and psychotic symptoms can occur in depression and schizophrenia, but no tests can differentiate these two problems. The case scenario also exemplifies other problems in today's psychiatric practice: lack of standardization of the diagnostic process, lack of communication between clinicians, lack of time to deal with people's most complex medical problems.

Sometimes it is said that when two psychiatrists examine the same patient, there will be two different diagnoses; when four psychiatrists examine the same patient, there will be four different diagnoses. Many factors contribute to this problem: patients' symptoms can change over time; patients can emphasize different problems to different doctors; doctors can use very different styles of interviewing to see what the patients' symptoms are; different physicians may have different diagnostic prototypes in mind; critical areas of pathology may not be explored. But the main reason is the fact that objective tests do not exist.

For years, I worked in a busy psychiatric emergency room. Patients would be interviewed first by a psychiatric clinician, a social worker or nurse, who then would present the patient's case to me. In turn, I would go into the examining room and interview the patient. Not infrequently, I got very different information, sometimes contradictory to the material obtained just a few minutes ago by the first clinician. Unless one starts to systematically study this phenomenon, including videotaping all interactions, it will never be entirely clear what causes these changes in information processing. But the fact that there are no objectively measurable findings, independent of the patient – physician relationship, is a major problem.

The bottom line is that there is no objective bench mark that can guide the diagnostic process in psychiatry. There is no way for psychiatrists to get feedback on their diagnostic work. In the next chapter, it will become clear why this is so problematic for the day to day psychiatric practice.

Where does this leave the field?

With the discovery of the first effective psychiatric medications, like chlorpromazine and imipramine, in the middle of the last century, a need arose for researchers to be able to more accurately identify patients suffering from the same mental illness. Also, progress through treatment needed to be measurable. When similar conditions can be identified by different investigators and progress can be measured, it is possible to study and replicate what medications benefit patients with a particular mental illness. Hence, diagnostic criteria for different psychiatric disorders were developed. Also, symptom ratings scales were designed to follow change over time during treatment. Eventually, these criteria culminated in a major revision of the official nomenclature of psychiatric diagnoses in the Diagnostic and Statistical Manual of Mental Disorders (DSM) by the American Psychiatric Association (APA). Recently, the publication of the latest version, DSM-5, has stirred up many debates, most of them having to do with the topic at hand: how are these diagnoses established without objective confirmation and who is right in establishing criteria? DSM-5 reaffirmed that biological measures are not yet part of the classification of mental disorders. In the early 1990's, it was hoped that, by the 21th century, we would have some chemical or imaging tests to strengthen our diagnostic abilities. But the complexities of the brain and its dysfunctions have proven too much for fast progress. So, the debate between critics and advocates of DSM-5 will continue and psychiatrists will be left without corrective feedback.

The fact remains that the DSM is likely the best psychiatry can do under the current circumstances. It does provide some degree of, at least, reliability, if not some face validity to the diagnostic prototypes and templates that physicians need to use to help their patients.

To enhance reliability in research, structured diagnostic interviews were developed, based on the diagnostic criteria of the DSM. These diagnostic instruments spell out what questions should be asked of the patient in exploring different areas of psychopathology. While many of these interviews are too lengthy to be used in clinical practice, in the past two decades, clinician friendly versions have been made available. They help the physician in making sure core symptoms of different disorders are explored.

Another development happened with the increased investigation of treatments for mental disorders, especially since the 1990's. Guidelines were developed on how to approach the management of depression, bipolar disorder, schizophrenia, post-traumatic stress disorder, conduct disorder, eating disorders and many others. Different professional organizations have contributed to this process. These guidelines are broad descriptions on how to approach the treatment of a particular psychiatric problem. They are based on the latest evidence from large controlled studies, naturalistic follow up data, epidemiological investigations and expert opinion. They are readily available for consultation to any practitioner.

So, the field has some tools available, albeit imperfect ones: diagnostic criteria, structured interviews, rating scales and treatment guidelines. It can be argued that, in the absence of objective data, the best clinical practice will result from using these tools at all times, while still individualizing the treatment for each particular patient.

But are these criteria, rating scales, structured interviews and guidelines utilized in the day to day practice of psychiatric medicine in academic centers, private practices and community clinics?

CHAPTER III: THE RESULT OF THE LACK OF CORRECTIVE FEEDBACK: LOSS OF

CRITICAL THINKING

When you take a test on a certain subject and you never get feedback on your results, you will never know if your answers were right or wrong. Moreover, when you retake the test, the chances that you will apply the same thinking process and make the same mistakes are high. If this process repeats itself over and over, you may lose interest and not care so much anymore about getting the right answers. At the same time, your cognitive skills are not being sharpened, because you are never challenged with the mistakes you make. Learning comes to a halt.

I believe this process is very applicable to psychiatry. Making a psychiatric diagnosis is like taking a test without feedback on the correctness of your answer to the question: from what mental illness is this patient suffering? Faced with this type of situation several times per day, diagnostic acumen and interest in getting it right diminish over time, unless specific precautions are taken. One could argue that the outcome of a particular treatment is some form of feedback in psychiatry. However, this argument is flawed for many reasons: many psychiatric conditions respond to placebo treatment; psychiatric medications are not disease specific but symptom specific and symptoms are shared between different illnesses; several medications treat more than one symptom, etc.

About 15 years ago, while working in a large hospital's psychiatric emergency room (ER), I noticed that inpatient attendings had a habit of making the same diagnoses regardless of the presenting problems of the patients. I noticed that attending A usually diagnosed patients with schizophrenia, while attending B usually diagnosed patients with bipolar disorder, mixed episode type, and so on.

As a matter of fact, when the same patient was admitted on different occasions, his or her diagnosis changed, despite presenting with similar signs and symptoms. It appeared that the only variable that changed was the treating attending physician to whom the patient happened to be assigned. One day, I asked an emergency room staff member to pick up ten medical records of patients who had recently been discharged from the hospital. I asked the staff member to reveal neither identifying nor clinical information, but only the discharge diagnosis, made by inpatient attendings. Eight out of the ten times, I correctly guessed the name of the inpatient attending who had discharged the patient.

How is this possible?

I wanted to make things better for the patients and easier for the attendings. I trained all staff, who evaluated patients in the emergency room prior to admission to the inpatient units, in the use of a structured interview. Core symptoms of disorders were identified, while negative findings were documented as well. Diagnoses were made according to inclusion and exclusion criteria, as outlined in the DSM. Staff were required to video or audiotape their interviews, with consent of the patients. This made it possible to give feedback to individual clinicians and increase the reliability of the diagnostic process in the emergency department. The findings were well documented in the emergency department's note, accompanying the patients to the unit.

After two years, this intensive effort in the emergency unit of the hospital had no effect whatsoever on the behavior of the inpatient attendings!

How is this possible?

These attendings were the test takers discussed in the beginning of this chapter. Over and over again, they took a test (diagnosing a patient) but never received feedback. Over the years, they lost interest in honing their skills, so much so, that when given a strategy to help them take the test, it no longer fazed them. Nobody ever challenged them on their repetitive labeling of serious mental health problems.

During a quiet moment in the ER, I picked up an old medical record of a patient discharged with a schizophrenia diagnosis. I read the inpatient attending's admission note, every daily physician note, and every single nursing and therapist note over a six day stay in an acute psychiatric unit. Not one positive (such as hallucinations, delusions, thought disorder, bizarre posturing) or negative symptom (such as flat affect, poverty of speech, poor motivation, social isolation) of schizophrenia was written down in the entire record. Upon what was the diagnosis based?

How is this possible?

I believe that many psychiatrists have lost their ability and / or motivation to critically think through a differential diagnostic process. They accept at face value what a patient complains about and, within minutes, come to a hasty conclusion about the underlying problem. Then, they institute a treatment accordingly. They almost never get feedback on their diagnostic conclusion. They almost never learn that their thinking was right or wrong. On occasion, feedback does occur: when a depressed patient is started on an antidepressant and becomes manic, the real diagnosis may have become apparent. But these instances are rare.

Making a correct diagnosis in medicine is difficult, especially in psychiatry. Many psychiatric problems manifest themselves mostly through subjective symptoms, not observable to others. Depressed mood, loss of interest, ruminations, worries, hallucinations, poor focus, suicidal thoughts are examples of psychiatric symptoms reported by patients without external validation. Objective signs, when present, are open to different interpretations: is poverty of speech a sign of depression or a negative symptom of a psychotic illness? Is rambling speech a sign of mania or schizophrenia? Is restlessness related to anxiety or ADHD? So, critical thinking is of utmost importance: complaints need to be put in the proper context; the possibility that problems with mood, behavior and thinking can be caused by general medical conditions needs to be kept in the forefront; the reality that signs and symptoms can belong to different conditions need to be entertained; historical data and current observations need to be integrated. Without feedback, this is a daunting task that is difficult but possible in most circumstances.

For example, when a patient presents with the chief complaint of auditory hallucinations, an attempt should be made to evaluate the authenticity of this complaint by having the patient describe the nature, quality, quantity, content and circumstances of the alleged perceptual disturbance. If the description matches known characteristics of auditory hallucinations, a differential diagnostic process is indicated. Is there evidence of a general medical or neurological condition related to the chief complaint? Is the patient using drugs? Does the patient report symptoms and show signs of a psychotic illness, or a mood disorder? This process is elaborate, time consuming and effortful. It requires diligence and energy. I believe that many psychiatrists have lost the motivation to go through it time and again.

CHAPTER IV: THE RESULT OF THE LOSS OF CRITICAL THINKING: DIAGNOSTIC

SLOPPINESS

In 2007, a study was published reporting that the diagnosis of pediatric bipolar disorder increased 40

times in the U.S. in the decade 1997 – 2007! When a condition increases over time in a given

population, several explanations are possible. One possibility is a true increase caused by genetic,

epigenetic, and /or environmental factors. Another possibility is the fact that the condition is

identified more frequently because of better diagnostic tools. Changes in diagnostic criteria may play

a role. Better treatment methods may draw more attention to the illness. However, it is extremely

unlikely that any of these factors can explain a 40 time increase in ten years. The interaction between

genetic and environmental influences is a very slow process, happening over many decades, if not

centuries. Other conditions have seen an increase in recognition based on better diagnostic or

treatment availability, but never such a rapid change in the frequency of the diagnostic label. And

other countries have not seen this dramatic rise in pediatric bipolar disorder. So what happened in

the U.S.?

I believe that the answer lies in diagnostic sloppiness. On a daily basis, in children and adults alike, I

see the diagnosis of bipolar disorder on patients' records without any supporting documentation.

When examined, these patients deny a history of core manic or hypomanic symptoms, an absolute

must for the diagnosis of bipolar disorder to be considered. They deny discrete episodes of mood

disturbance or cycles of depressive and manic periods. Many of them report quick irritability,

explosiveness and impulsive aggression. Many times, these problems are reported as part of ongoing attention deficit hyperactivity disorder (ADHD), conduct disorder, substance use, depression, or personality disorders. But many psychiatrists no longer take the time and make the effort to elicit a history of core manic symptoms or discrete mood cycles. As soon as someone reports explosiveness or "mood swings" (meaning quick irritability), the label of bipolar disorder is attached.

During a one month period, I examined 16 patients who were recently released from a prison mental health system. Thirteen patients had a bipolar disorder diagnosis written on their transfer papers. Upon examination and careful questioning to elicit manic symptoms, one patient identified clear manic episodes and one patient appeared to have had hypomanic episodes in the past. The other 11 patients denied ever experiencing manic symptoms as described in any diagnostic system such as the DSM. Even purely statistically speaking, it would be extremely unlikely that 13 out of 16 patients suffered from bipolar disorder. Other conditions, such as depression, personality disorders, or ADHD, are more prevalent. Two patients commented on the problem themselves by stating they did not believe the diagnosis. One of them proclaimed: "I know I am not bipolar because I have never been manic!"

This "bipolar problem" is entirely an American phenomenon. It is so pervasive that many patients become addicted to their "bipolar": "my bipolar is acting up", "I am bipolar", "I was diagnosed bipolar, and so that's what I am". Patients become defensive, sometimes outraged, when an explanation is provided that they do not report a history consistent with this illness. They want the label.

In 2011, I published a commentary with the following title: "Poor practice, managed care, and a magic pill society: Have we created a mental health monster" (Psychiatric Times; volume 28, 2, 2011). The mental health monster mentioned in the title is exactly the tremendous bipolar disorder overdiagnosis. In this commentary, I described how poor psychiatric practice, combined with pressures from insurance companies, play into a society where people want a quick fix, do not want to take responsibility for their health, and want a label to blame for their problems in life. It is indeed easier to take pills, rather than to learn skills. In many situations, it is also advantageous monetarily: the chances that the U.S. disability system will pay for a bipolar label are higher than the chances it will pay for an ADHD diagnosis, for example. But where does the buck stop?

19

It should stop with psychiatrists. The differentiation from other conditions and the identification of true bipolar disorder is often a difficult and lengthy process. The problem, however, is the fact that many psychiatrists don't even try to do a better job. The test takers have given up; it no longer matters; who is right anyway; many people want the diagnostic label. Diagnostic sloppiness is exemplified beyond belief in the American bipolar disorder phenomenon.

Many other diagnoses are undergoing the same fate. Take post-traumatic stress disorder (PTSD), for example. Again, specific criteria should be used to justify the diagnosis, among them a severe traumatic incident and symptoms related to the present re-living of the past trauma. However, in practice, many patients are diagnosed with PTSD without reporting any re-living symptomatology whatsoever. Research has clearly shown that only a minority of significantly traumatized people develop the specific syndrome of PTSD. Clearly, past trauma can lead to other mental health problems, but diagnostic differentiation is needed to better guide the treatment.

A third example is adult ADHD. Attention deficit hyperactivity disorder starts in childhood. Symptoms are present during the elementary school ages. It certainly can continue to cause impairment into adult years. But adult ADHD is frequently misdiagnosed, mostly as bipolar disorder, sometimes as an anxiety problem. Restlessness, low frustration tolerance and quick irritability are quite common in adults with ADHD, but there are no discrete episodes of manic symptoms. At other times, ADHD is over diagnosed. Adults who claim to have ADHD symptoms are often not questioned about their childhood problems; corroborating information is not obtained, and the patients are not examined for other conditions that may cause concentration problems. They leave the office with a prescription for stimulants! Diagnostic sloppiness can indeed lead to either over or under diagnosis.

One hallmark of this diagnostic sloppiness is the acceptance of the patient's statements at face value. When a patient says, "I have bipolar disorder", there is frequently no attempt made to evaluate the accuracy of this statement. I see many evaluations stating: "The patient has been diagnosed with bipolar disorder. The patient is currently…" The diagnosis is unconditionally accepted and treatment is continued or changed based on this presumption. No critical thinking, analysis, or evaluation is done. When a patient claims to "hear voices", many times no attempt is made to critically evaluate this complaint: is the report consistent with what we know about auditory hallucinations or is something else going on. When a patient reports "anxiety", all too often the prescription pad comes out to write for benzodiazepines without a necessary assessment of what the patient is experiencing.

When a patient changes clinicians in other disciplines of medicine, there is usually a trail of objective tests, such as blood work and x-rays, that accompanies the patient and guides the new clinician in providing continuity of care. This is not the case in psychiatry. Every new patient, no matter what diagnosis they report from previous doctors, should be examined with a critical mind. When this is not done, the diagnostic sloppiness is being perpetuated.

CHAPTER V: THE RESULT OF DIAGNOSTIC SLOPPINESS: POOR DOCUMENTATION

Medical record documentation is extremely important for many reasons. In most situations, it is the only tangible evidence of the encounter between the patient and the physician. Especially in psychiatry, a specialty without objective test results, documentation, for the most part, represents the entire examination. The medical record becomes the vehicle through which care is provided by the same clinician over time. It also serves a communication function between different doctors. Among other purposes of the medical record system are quality improvements and risk management.

In essence, the medical record needs to provide an opportunity to retrospectively review the patient's complaints and condition, the examinations performed and the physician's thinking process. Diagnoses should be substantiated by descriptions of symptoms, their onset, duration, severity and impairment. Negative findings should be clarified as well. The record needs to state the treatment that was initiated and the recommendations and education that were provided to the patient. Follow up notes need to specify the outcome of the treatment and any adjustments that were made. All of this should be done in a legible and professional manner.

Now let's take a look at the nature of documentation I have encountered over the years. Let me begin with the most absurd and incomprehensible example, although it is, by far, not the only one of its kind that I have encountered. The following paragraph is the beginning of the history of present illness in a psychiatric evaluation that was signed electronically, which means it cannot be changed or corrected. It also means that this physician agrees with this document as the final and official version. In addition, it means that this record can be sent to other physicians, health care providers, upon consent of the patient. Here it is:

"Don't Fred was for facts. Me running cannot see screen go answer due to of time. A machine thing now because economic numbers mean dependent or he Patient presents for a psychiatric evaluation."

I like to emphasize again that this is an official document that represents this physician's work!

How is this possible?

Even though I could give you an explanation of how this came about, the explanation doesn't matter. What matters is that this physician signed off on this record, indicating that this represents the final version of his work and encounter with the patient. Can you imagine being a primary care physician, a therapist, a lawyer, reading this history as the representation of this doctor's clinical work?

What is happening here? Where is the accountability? Where are the professional and ethical standards?

Documentation needs to reflect one's clinical acumen, differential diagnostic skills, concern for the patient's wellbeing, and the treatment plan. But if you clearly don't care what your documentation looks like, how can you say you care about the patient, the diagnosis and the treatment? After all, the record is the only concrete evidence of the encounter.

A record should start with identifying information of the patient, which should include the patient's age, race, marital status, family members living with the patient, and employment status. The following example shows the identifying/demographic section of a signed record:

"presented here due to a diagnosis of depression and had been seen in the past and has been without treatment for a year--mood problems"

What happened here? Who is this patient? What is the patient's age, or race, or marital status? Is this patient identified by depression?

Again, this record reflects this physician's work.

Let's continue with some more shocking findings. The history of present illness section in a psychiatric evaluation is supposed to contain some essential pieces of information: how the evaluation was performed and if any specific tools were used (like structured interviews); the main findings such as symptoms and syndromes that justify the diagnoses; the duration of the problems; symptom rating scales; the normal findings; a risk/safety assessment in terms of suicidal or aggressive behavior; the patient's impairment and level of functioning. The following two pages show one evaluation from my records compared to a total history of present illness section from another doctor:

The patient was examined with a review of core symptoms (DSM-IV) of depression, mania, psychosis, substance use, GAD, OCD, PTSD, social phobia, panic disorder, ADHD, disruptive behavior disorders, eating disorders. The Mini International Neuropsychiatric Interview was administered.

Co-lateral information was obtained from: clinic records /

...Chief Complaint: "depression"

...Reported SYNDROMES/SYMPTOMS are consistent with:

* depression: in 2005, low mood, anger, loss of interest, fluctuating sleep, low appetite x 2 y / no suicidality / remission did occur / currently, similar problems but also anxiety and poor focus / no suicidality / no mania / no psychosis /

...Clinical Global Impression-SEVERITY Scale (1=normal, 2=borderline, 3=mild, 4=moderate, 5=moderately severe, 6=severe, 7=catastrophic): 4

...SYMPTOM RATING SCALES:

PHQ-9, a depression rating scale: 20 / 27, indicating moderately severe depression;
R.A.F.F.T., a screen for substance use: 1 item endorsed, low likelihood for substance use disorder;
Standardized Assessment of Personality-Abbreviated Scale: 4 / 8, good likelihood for a personality disorder;
PANSS items (1=absent-7=extreme): Delusions: 1 ; Conceptual Disorganization: 1 ; Hallucinatory Behavior: 1 ; Blunted Affect: 1 ; Emotional Withdrawal: 1 ; Poor Rapport: 1 . Total score: 6 ;
Global Assessment of Functioning Scale: 52

...Reported DURATION of symptoms is 1 year

..IMPAIRMENT due to psychiatric symptoms: the following functional adaptations are impaired: neuro-vegetative functioning; social relatedness;

...There is NO EVIDENCE FOR mania, GAD, panic, OCD, PTSD, social phobia, psychosis, substance use, PDD, tics, ADHD, Conduct disorder, eating disorders.

...Reported STRESSORS are pain. Reported SUPPORTS are parents.

...Identified RISK/PROTECTIVE FACTORS FOR DANGEROUS (SUICIDAL/AGGRESSIVE) BEHAVIOR are: depression, intermittent insomnia / Nature of previous suicide attempts: none ///
No current hopelessness, SI, SIB, HI, substance use, psychosis, interpersonal aggressivity. No access to weapons. No history of suicide attempts. Mother of dependent children.
Risk assessment: low /

Before the past summer --no evidence of any symptoms

My record is not perfect. Everyone has his or her own style of documenting information. I prefer a style in which information is clearly divided in different sections and described in piecemeal fashion, rather than a long text with full sentences. Upon my review during the next visit with the patient, it allows me to focus on the important information in an efficient manner. But what is the style of the other physician?

This, once again, represents the entire section of the bulk of the psychiatric evaluation, and, as such, represents this physician's work!

It happens quite often that I see an entire history of present illness consist of quotes by the patient, such as: "I am stressed out"; "I hear voices telling me to kill myself"; "I can't stand being around people". There is no evaluative quality in the document, no interpretation of signs and symptoms, and no referral to any cohesive syndrome. Anyone could listen to someone and record what they say!

In a record I received from a psychiatrist on the West Coast, the following paragraph was the entire history of present illness:

Completed inpatient rehab in 2008 and again in 2010. Has mood swings: happy – angry – happy – angry. Became aggressive, after age 19.

At the end of this document, the diagnosis was spelled out as bipolar disorder! Based on this history of present illness, not one diagnosis can be assigned to this patient's problems. A diagnosis of bipolar disorder requires the documentation of at least one manic episode with core manic symptoms for a minimum of one week, leading to significant impairment. The possibility of a substance induced mood disorder in this patient certainly exists and needs to be addressed in the evaluation. None of this was done, while the patient was prescribed a mood stabilizer, with significant weight gain as a result.

In 2013, I published a brief article: "Better psychiatric documentation: from SOAP to PROMISE" (Current Psychiatry, March 2013, Pearls). It gives an outline for documenting follow up visits that is easy to remember and covers the most important facts that should be in a note. I have distributed the article to several clinics but, so far, have not seen any interest in it.

Considering the above examples, what is happening in the psychiatric field? The test takers have given up, not only in trying to get the right answer, but also in trying to fill in all the bubbles on the answering sheet. One could argue that a clinician could do an excellent job in the examination of the patient, yet document poorly. That is certainly a possibility, but I do not believe it is a common occurrence. In general, documentation reflects the overall quality of the encounter. A physician who is thoughtful, caring, and up to date in knowledge will generally write a note that is comprehensive in its scope.

I believe that the above examples of problems with documentation are the result of diagnostic sloppiness and the absence of critical thinking, stemming from the lack of corrective feedback. These physicians did not go through a differential diagnostic process, and, as such, did not document much. They had no tests to comment on and had lost the motivation to describe their interpretation of the subjective symptoms and objective signs presented by the patient.

How would the medical community look upon a surgeon's note stating: "I opened and closed the patient"?

CHAPTER VI: PHYSICIAN RELATED FACTORS CONTRIBUTING TO THE PROBLEM

Besides the loss of critical thinking and diagnostic sloppiness, there are other factors contributing to the current state of affairs in psychiatric practice: not following evidence based treatment guidelines and lack of continuing medical education (CME).

Recently, I discussed a case with a colleague at a major university in New York. A young patient had been admitted for severe psychosis for a second time in a short period. The patient had been started on risperidone, for schizophrenia, during his first admission. He did respond to the medication but stopped taking it soon after his discharge. He relapsed and was readmitted. My colleague told me that the patient was discharged from his second admission on haloperidol decanoate, a long acting injectable antipsychotic, and risperidone pills. Why haloperidol and why two antipsychotics? There is not one guideline or one schizophrenia expert who would recommend this action. The logical treatment would have been long acting injectable risperidone. The patient had responded to risperidone pills but stopped taking them. An injectable form has a higher chance that the patient would receive the treatment he needs. But why change to haloperidol? And why prescribe two antipsychotics? There is no evidence that antipsychotic poly-pharmacy in a person with new onset schizophrenia is more effective. As a matter of fact, the chance that this patient will experience more side effects is a lot higher, again increasing the possibility of his stopping the treatment. Neither evidence based treatment nor any guidelines, of which there are several for schizophrenia treatment, were followed in this case. And this happened at a tertiary care psychiatric hospital.

I regularly see patients who have been prescribed two antidepressants in the same family of medications or two antidepressants in related families. There is some evidence that the use of two antidepressants at the same time may be more helpful under certain conditions. However, the evidence points to antidepressants with different working mechanisms, not medications with the same or related mechanisms of action. And yet, I regularly see patients prescribed two serotonin re-uptake inhibitors (SSRI) at the same time, or an SSRI and a serotonin – norepinephrine re-uptake inhibitor (SNRI). There is no literature on the effectiveness and, more important, on the safety of this approach. Similar problems with not following evidence based medicine are apparent in the following scenarios: prescribing two benzodiazepines at the same time; prescribing controlled substances to patients with addiction problems; prescribing certain anticonvulsants for mood stabilization even though studies have shown they are no better than placebo; prescribing atypical antipsychotics for insomnia.

The problem of not following evidence guidelines is closely related to the problem of not pursuing enough continuing medical education. Over the years, I have discussed psychiatric treatments with physicians all over the nation. It becomes clear quite quickly that many physicians are up to date with the latest findings and studies, but it is also very noticeable that many are not. Medicine is a never ending learning experience, not only through seeing many patients and their responses to treatment, but also by continuing to restore and increase the memory bank of findings reported in the literature. This requires reading a few hours per week. In this regard, the requirement of state medical boards for physicians to engage in 50 hours of CME per year is entirely insufficient for two reasons: it is not enough and it is not enforced in any credible fashion. The requirement is enforced through an honor system. But do physicians who care so little about their work, as manifested by their documentation, care about furthering their education? Many psychiatrists do care, but too many apparently do not.

CHAPTER VII: NON-PHYSICIAN FACTORS CONTRIBUTING TO THE PROBLEM

It is my opinion that psychiatrists are solely responsible for the current state of psychiatric practice. The problems with the lack of critical thinking, diagnostic sloppiness and poor documentation are totally in the realm of the individual physician's behavior. But other factors are contributing, sometimes directly and sometimes in reaction to the problems.

Insurance Companies

Even though they use the term "managed care ", it is very apparent by their behavior that insurance companies only manage cost. And they have significantly contributed to creating a "mental health monster", as I pointed out in "Poor practice, managed care, and a magic pill society: Have we created a mental health monster" (Psychiatric Times volume 28, 2, 2011). Many times, insurance companies do not pay for specific treatments unless a certain diagnosis is given, even though the evidence base in the medical literature would support the treatment. In psychiatry, without objective test findings, diagnoses are easily manipulated. Remember the 40 times increase in the pediatric bipolar diagnosis between 1997 and 2007. Part of this problem is driven by insurance companies only paying for certain treatments when there is a "severe" diagnosis, such as bipolar disorder. These treatments may range from medications, to intensive behavioral treatments, to hospitalizations. When a patient is very irritable, impulsive and explosive, and requires a medication to help with self control, but the insurance company is denying the medication unless a bipolar disorder diagnosis is present, this will be a factor contributing to the diagnostic sloppiness. It reinforces the psychiatrist's hasty use of the bipolar diagnosis. When a patient presents to an emergency room and is in need of psychiatric hospitalization to ensure safety to self or others, insurance companies will only agree to cover the admission financially with a severe diagnosis, like a psychotic illness or bipolar disorder. When an insurance company only reimburses for an evaluation done in one visit, and does not reimburse for an evaluation over several sessions, it reinforces diagnostic sloppiness. For coding and

31

billing purposes, the clinician will need to provide a diagnosis at the end of one examination. In some circumstances, it doesn't leave much time to explore in detail the differential diagnostic questions at hand, or to use state of the art diagnostic tools, like structured interviews.

I still remember the day, years ago, when, in a span of one hour, the same insurance company denied two medications for two patients. Medication A was denied for the first patient because it was not indicated by the Food and Drug Administration (FDA) for the patient's condition, even though there was evidence based literature of its use in exactly that condition. Medication B was denied for the second patient, despite a FDA indication for that patient's diagnosis! The insurance company stated that another generic medication needed to be tried even though this medication had no FDA approval for any condition in this patient's age group! Insurance companies use anything and everything they can to reduce their costs without regard to the patient's care. In psychiatry, where objective tests do not exist, it reinforces diagnostic sloppiness.

And, if insurance companies truly cared about managing the care provided to the patient, why do they pay for evaluations that are documented in the manner described in a previous chapter?

Lawyers and the Disability System

It is sometimes said that the American disability system is a mental health system. Because of the absence of objective tests, it sometimes appears that a psychiatric diagnosis can be pulled out of a hat. Many disability lawyers send their clients to psychiatrists to get a mental health diagnosis. It is easier to claim that someone can't work because of depression, anxiety, or psychosis, than to claim that a general medical problem exists. A physical health problem would need to be substantiated by a blood test, or an imaging study. I clearly recall a phone call I received from a lawyer representing one of my patients in a disability appeal. My evaluation, which was released to the lawyer with the patient's consent, stated that there was no impairment in vegetative functioning, activities of daily living, memory and understanding, concentration and pace, and social relatedness. These different areas of functioning are considered by the social security administration's adjudicators in determining eligibility for benefits. The lawyer asked me to delete the sentence, stating there was no impairment, from the evaluation!

I recently saw a young man for an evaluation. He claimed to be hearing hallucinatory voices. Hallucinations are a totally subjective experience for which we have no objective test available in the clinic setting. However, this patient's description was very atypical, compared to the descriptions I have heard many times from patients suffering from severe mental illnesses. Also, the patient showed no other signs at all of a psychiatric disturbance: he was well related with normal activity level, normal eye contact, normal affect, normal speech, and normal thought process. At the end of the evaluation, he presented papers from a lawyer, asking me to rate his level of impairment in different areas of functioning. Was this patient having hallucinations without any other sign of a psychiatric disturbance or was he malingering? Would a psychiatrist in private practice, being dependent on a patient's return to sustain his or her business, feel free to put down such a response? Would a psychiatrist in a clinic setting be prepared for a confrontation with the patient about what is really going on? Or is a psychiatrist's diagnostic sloppiness, by accepting at face value what the patient says, being reinforced by the system? By diagnosing the patient with a psychosis, the patient and the lawyer will be satisfied and may return.

Magic Pill Society

As a child psychiatrist, I encounter more situations where I need to say to a parent that medications are not appropriate for their child, than situations where I need to convince a reluctant parent that medication should be part of the treatment. Parents give me a harder time stopping medication for their children, compared to starting pharmacotherapy. The same happens with adult patients. I regularly see patients who complain of depression but whose problem is clearly related to their maladaptive coping style or their frustrations with life, not clinical depression. But when taken at face value, they are diagnosed with depression and prescribed an antidepressant. Patients and families want a quick and easy fix to any problem. They do not want to work in psychotherapy, change their lifestyle, exercise, modify their sleep habits, or quit their substance use to target their problems. They want a pill. And by accepting their complaints, expressed in psychiatric jargon, without critical thinking, physicians are giving them their wish: a medication. And the psychiatrists are doing their job, or are they?

This diagnostic sloppiness has given rise to an entitlement in certain patients, never seen before.

33

They speak psychiatric jargon and demand certain treatments. They complain of anxiety and demand benzodiazepines. They claim to have ADHD and demand stimulants. They claim to hear voices and demand a disability statement. Upon careful examination, they either do not substantiate the claim, or become defensive and, at times, outright hostile. But diagnostic sloppiness may satisfy their desires, and reinforces their behavior. The psychiatrist, in the mean time, does not have to engage in the difficult process of differential diagnosis or confrontation with the patient. And feedback is not available, so who cares?

CHAPTER VIII: SUMMARY OF THE PROBLEM AND THE CONSEQUENCES FOR PATIENTS AND SOCIETY

Psychiatry is a unique medical specialty: it deals with the most complex organ in the body and with the most intricate human qualities of emotions, thinking and behavior. And yet, it has no objective way to confirm its findings.

I believe that the lack of objective validation of mental illnesses, in combination with many other factors, has created a critically diseased state of the practice of American psychiatry: diagnostic sloppiness.

With society on an accelerating pace, the internet explaining every imaginable symptom or syndrome, lawyers and insurance companies intruding in medical practice like never before, people feeling ever more entitled to whatever they desire, psychiatrists should firmly adhere to the state of the science and art of practicing their medical specialty. Instead, many physicians do not keep up with their field, fold under the pressure of time and patients' attitudes, and have abandoned the ultimate tool in medicine: differential diagnostic thinking. Poor, inadequate and insufficient documentation reveals the dark side of this disease.

The consequences are manifold. The most important one is the fact that many patients do not get the appropriate treatment for their condition. Patients are prescribed the wrong medication. Others are prescribed medication but should have other treatments instead. Providing the wrong treatment will prolong the patient's suffering.

Several classes of psychiatric medications have serious side effects, such as weight gain, metabolic changes, cardiovascular risks, or blood related problems. Patients taking these medications for the wrong reason are exposed to these side effects, while the benefits are doubtful. Psychiatrists do not need to add to the epidemic of obesity in this country by prescribing weight inducing medications without a well thought out rationale. Prescribing weight inducing antipsychotics for sleep or for ADHD misdiagnosed as bipolar disorder is inappropriate but rampant. Prescribing two medications of the same family poses unnecessary risks to the patient and cost to society.

Society is paying for this diagnostic sloppiness which leads to inappropriate treatments. Healthcare is tremendously expensive in this country but clearly not of higher quality compared to many other developed nations. Disability payments are higher in this country as well. I believe that many patients with psychiatric disabilities can productively contribute to society, but instead receive a monthly disability check. Psychiatric diagnostic sloppiness makes this possible.

Insurance companies are clamming down more and more because of inappropriate prescribing practices and escalating costs. But their increased intrusiveness is adding to the problem, not alleviating it.

Patients' entitlements are reinforced by diagnostic sloppiness and create other problems: abuse and diversion of prescription pills is at record highs. Diagnostic sloppiness leads to inappropriate prescribing of controlled substances as well.

Psychiatric disorders are seriously disabling conditions. Diagnosing them, including drawing the line between normal and abnormal functioning, is many times quite difficult. Treatments are far from ideal in terms of effectiveness and safety. Individuals, families, and society are paying an enormous emotional and financial toll. All of this should spur a tremendous effort by psychiatric professionals to do the best job possible. Instead, American psychiatric practice has deteriorated and is facing a serious crisis. Already, many primary care physicians don't know where to turn for advice and consultation for their patients with mental illness.

CHAPTER IX: WHAT IS THE SOLUTION?

Several years ago, I attended a presentation about a stimulant medication administered by way of a patch applied to the skin. When the presenter discussed potential adverse events related to the cardiovascular system, a psychiatrist raised the question whether or not the patch could be applied to the chest area! Was this psychiatrist truly thinking that attaching the patch on the chest near the heart would give any more problems than when attached to the hip? I believe that an intelligent sixth grader could answer that question. But a medical doctor, who graduated high school, college, medical school and four years of residency, raising this question? So is part of the solution attracting smarter people into psychiatry? The truth is that most top medical students choose other specialties. Stigma, the financial burden of student loans, the length of training, poor modeling of cognitive skills by psychiatric mentors in medical schools, the lack of procedures, the lack of objective tests, lead many good students away from psychiatry.

Once physicians enter a psychiatric residency, the large majority of their time is spent with attending psychiatrists, many of whom show signs of the disease of psychiatric practice: diagnostic sloppiness. I was stunned, when I was supervising fifth year pediatric psychiatry fellows in a world renowned research institution, to learn that they had never seen a structured psychiatric interview. Is psychiatric residency becoming a scenario of the blind leading the blind? A standardization of training requirements and the reinforcement of its implementation could make some difference. But how have other requirements faired? Let's take a look at one example. Psychiatric residency programs have the requirement of teaching several types of psychotherapy, to the point of competency. As I am a member of the Academy of Cognitive Therapy, I volunteered several years ago to supervise residents for their cognitive therapy treatment of patients. The two residents that were assigned to me over two years were not able to present even one patient for supervision: the program did not assign them any cases! So much for implementing and reinforcing requirements!

Up until the middle 1990s, psychiatrists who were board certified had no official obligation, other than documenting 50 hours of CME per year, to maintain their status. Fortunately, this is changing. Currently, board certifications are only valid for ten years. Every ten years, a psychiatrist needs to fulfill several requirements to maintain certification. Among these are self assessment exercises, chart reviews according to certain guidelines, development of improvement plans based on the chart reviews, obtaining feedback from peers and patients, and a standardized written examination. I believe this is a step in the right direction, but I also believe the impact will be extremely limited. Let's review some of the requirements. Self assessment exercises are tests followed by a review of the answers by way of references in the literature. There is no pass or fail attached to it. Chart reviews are done by the physician on his or her own charts without external input. Peer reviews may boil down to, once again, the blind leading the blind: would someone in the same practice be honest and criticize a peer with whom they have daily contact? And it is well known that passing a written examination has little bearing on putting the knowledge into practice.

So, it is far from clear what needs to happen to turn around the prognosis of the diseased American psychiatric practice.

Attracting the brightest medical students appears out of reach. Improving training experiences seems more attainable, but the experience so far has not been encouraging at all. More oversight of practicing psychiatrists is an absolute must, but a nightmare in terms of implementation.

One could argue that it is the current generation of psychiatrists creating the problem, but this generation is training the next!

Another argument makes the case for "fee for performance" rather than "fee for service". In other words, physicians would be reimbursed according to their outcomes, not for just performing a procedure, like a psychiatric evaluation. But in a specialty without objective tests, this appears to be very difficult. We know that almost all mental illnesses, as we currently conceptualize them, are very heterogeneous in nature and are probably composed of different diseases with different treatment responses and prognoses. But we don't know how to separate them. This is a major obstacle in measuring outcomes between different clinicians or clinics.

Without objective feedback, test takers will be left in the dark. Some will make sure that they continue to approach the test with new knowledge and skills, but many will lose interest in doing so. Maybe teaching them more knowledge and skills before taking the test will help.

CHAPTER X: THE MOST RADICAL SOLUTION: THE ELIMINATION OF PSYCHIATRY AS
A PRIMARY MEDICAL SPECIALTY

If one believes, as I do, that the following etiological sequence, from lack of objective findings to loss of critical thinking to diagnostic sloppiness, is correct, then the earliest intervention in this sequence could be the most successful. While objective confirmation of mental illness remains a goal for the future, the loss of critical thinking can be resolved now.

I believe that psychiatry as a primary medical specialty should be abandoned and relegated to being a subspecialty of pediatrics for child psychiatry and a subspecialty of internal medicine for adult psychiatry. The path to becoming a psychiatrist would be the same as for becoming a cardiologist, a rheumatologist or a gastroenterologist. Psychiatrists would spend three years in internal medicine or pediatrics, subjected to corrective feedback, and supervised by attending medical specialists. Their thinking would be shaped and fine tuned before entering a two or three year subspecialty, psychiatry. Together with ongoing requirements to maintain board certification, I believe this has the best chance to improving the prognosis of American psychiatric practice. Many critics will say that there is already a shortage of psychiatrists and that this pathway will increase that shortage. But does the U.S. want numerous psychiatrists doing a lousy job or fewer psychiatrists doing a good job in treating the significantly mentally ill? I believe that the institution of good differential diagnostic thinking in psychiatry, together with a reorganization of how medicine is practiced, will not lead to more of a deficit in the number of psychiatrists, but will lead to much better quality of care. Pilot projects of integrated care show promising results. In these programs, psychiatrists take on the role of consultants to primary care physicians who treat the patients for their medical and psychiatric problems. Fewer psychiatrists are needed in these systems of care.

Psychiatry is an exciting medical specialty. Research is slowly gaining ground in unraveling the mysteries of the brain. At some point in the future, psychiatry will be on par with other medical specialties, and will rely on genetic testing, neuro-imaging, and chemical analyses to guide diagnosis and treatment. Psychiatrists better be prepared!

ABOUT THE AUTHOR

Leo Bastiaens, MD, earned his medical degree at the Catholic University of Leuven in Leuven, Belgium. He completed a residency in Psychiatry at Mount Sinai Medical Center in New York, and a fellowship in Child and Adolescent Psychiatry at McLean Hospital/Harvard University. He studied cognitive therapy at The Cleveland Center for Cognitive Therapy. He is certified by the American Board of Psychiatry and Neurology in Psychiatry and Child and Adolescent Psychiatry, and he is a certified member of The Academy of Cognitive Therapy. Dr. Bastiaens is Clinical Associate Professor of Psychiatry at the University Of Pittsburgh School Of Medicine. He has published numerous articles in peer-reviewed journals and has presented on a variety of psychiatric topics at national and international meetings.

www.ingramcontent.com/pod-product-compliance
Lightning Source LLC
Chambersburg PA
CBHW021047180526
45163CB00005B/2321